Fighting the Invincible

Fighting the Invincible

A caregiver's narrative of life with Parkinson's disease

Dr. Rajat Gupta (PT)

Suravi Sharan

Self-Published and Printed

828/6 Indira Nagar,

Dehradun-248006 (Uttrakhand)

India.

+91-7895167765

suravi2410@gmail.com

First Edition, 2024

ISBN: 978-93-340-6586-2

In the loving memory of Dr. Sarita

For

All the patients and caregivers

Disclaimer

This information is intended for educational purposes only and should not be construed as medical advice.

Parkinson's disease is a complex neurological condition, and treatment plans should be individualized based on each patient's specific needs and medical history. The information presented in this book is based on personal experiences and extensive research by the authors. However, it is not a substitute for professional medical care.

Always consult with a qualified healthcare professional for diagnosis, treatment recommendations, and answers to any questions you may have regarding Parkinson's disease.

The authors and publisher disclaim any and all liability for any damages arising directly or indirectly from the use of the information contained in this book.

We encourage you to stay informed about the latest research and treatment options for Parkinson's disease by consulting with your doctor and reputable medical organizations.

Preface

Parkinson's disease is a progressive neurodegenerative disorder that finds mention in the list of diseases of old age. However, it is no longer a disease of retirement. In recent years a lot of young people have also reported the occurrence of the disease.

It is the second-most common neurodegenerative disease after Alzheimer's, affecting over 8.5 million[1] people worldwide. In the United States alone, there are over 500,000 people living with Parkinson's disease, and this number is expected to double by 2040.

In India, the prevalence of the disease is lower than in other countries, but the sheer size of the population means that there are still an estimated 7 million[2] people living with Parkinson's disease. Most of these patients live in rural areas, where access to healthcare is limited. In addition, there are only around 1,200[3] neurologists in India, and only a handful of these specialize in movement disorders. The disease makes the patients dependent on other people, thereby making the role of caregivers essential.

Caregivers provide physical, emotional, and logistical support to their loved ones. As the disease progresses, the role of caregivers also changes. Experts have predicted a staggering 200-300% increase[4] in

---

[1] WHO. 2022. Launch of WHO's Parkinson disease technical brief
[2] Behari, Madhuri. Experiences of Parkinson's disease in India. The Lancet.
[3] Khadilkar, SV. Neurology in India. NIH
[4] Hussain, Farheen. Experts warn of 200-300% rise in Parkinson's in next few decades.TNN

Parkinson's disease cases in the next few decades. This means that it is imperative that we understand the nature of this disease and the behavior of its patients.

I got the opportunity to observe a caregiver for Parkinson's disease in 2017. That person was none other than my father, who was caring for his sister. Back then, little did I know that I would become one such caregiver one day. On observation, I discovered that the task was extremely daunting. As the patient with Parkinson's disease faces difficulty in all the domains of life, they require assistance.

This book has been written after meticulous observation of the patient's behavior, consultations with the neurologist, online research and experiences of other caregivers. This book aims to raise awareness about the disease and provide hope and support. It is dedicated to making the journey easier for both the patient and the caregiver.

20 April. 24   Suravi Sharan

Contents

Chapter 1- Prisoners of the body and the mind

Helplessly trapped in one's own body that shows involuntary movement of limbs ultimately leading to complete inactivity/overactivity of body and a disturbed mind.

In his ground-breaking book "An Essay on Shaking Palsy", James Parkinson has mentioned tremors to be the defining signs of the disease. However, he has further mentioned that the onset of the disease is with *"slight sense of weakness with proneness to trembling in some particular parts, sometimes in the head and most commonly in the arms and the legs[5]"*.

The disease begins with a flicker, silently like a whisper in the stillness. The hesitation in the gait goes unnoticeable till the time it reaches a stage where the stiffness becomes visible in posture. The most agonizing consequence of this disease is

---

[5] Parkinson, James. (1817) *An Essay on Shaking Palsy.*

the relentless stripping of not only control, but also of independence of doing the things they love. The patients rely greatly on the caregivers for things as small as a brush against the teeth. While the first tremors are mere shimmers, the disease culminates in a ruthless choreographer, disrupting the delicate balance of the body.

It is a chronic disease i.e. it is persistent and shows long lasting effects. As per the research, the patients tend to live with the disease for 10-20 years after the diagnosis. It is considered to be a disorder in which the motor system of the central nervous system (CNS) gets affected. The motor system supports movements and reflexes. Thus, a person with the disorder faces difficulty in voluntary movement. As the disease advances, various other cognitive, behavioural, sensory and psychological changes may occur.

The usual onset of the disease generally occurs above the age of 60yrs. Age increases the risk of Parkinson's and therefore as the age of the population increases, the risk of more people suffering from the disease increases. However, over the years, young patients have also been diagnosed with the disease. Patients as young as 29 years as well as below have been diagnosed with the disease. In most Western countries, late-onset Parkinson's disease is more commonly reported, while in countries like Japan, early-onset Parkinson's disease appears to be more frequent. In Young Onset Parkinson's Disease, the symptoms of the disease can be observed between 21-40 years of age. If the disease occurs below 21 years of age then it is called Juvenile parkinsonism[6] and it occurs rarely.

The disorder can get worse if treatment is not provided at an appropriate time. However, it does not directly cause death, instead it puts strain on the body which leads to the development of life-threatening diseases. Patients with Parkinson's disease can manage their condition with more ease if quality care is provided.

From the shadows of history

James Parkinson documented his study in 1817 but the disease also finds mention in Ayurveda where it is referred to as Kampavata (where "kampa" means tremor in Sanskrit).

It is mentioned in Charak Samhita which is one of the oldest and the most authoritative texts of Ayurveda. The chapter on major diseases entitled as "Maharoga Adhyaya" mentions "vepathu" which means "shaking" or "trembling". Vepathu comes under the category of Nanatmaja Vyadhi that are the endogenous diseases caused by individual doshas. It was 7th century when physician Madhava described Vepathu as "sarvang kampa" i.e. the feeling of whole-body tremor and "shirokampa" i.e. head tremor.

------

[6] Parkinsonism is a condition that occurs when a person has symptoms and brain dysfunction commonly associated with Parkinson's disease but also has other symptoms related to an additional condition or cause.

4

Vepathu was replaced by "kampavata" in the 12th century AD.

In 175 AD, the keen eye of Galen, a Roman physician, meticulously documented the tremor that fostered in stillness. He also mentioned the bowed posture and the paralysis that cast a chilling shadow across movement.

During the 18th century, an authentic book of Ayurvedic medicine was written by Kaviraj Govinda Das Sen namely Bhaishajya Ratnavali. It described various diseases, their treatments and dietary requirements. He mentioned "Kampavata" and its symptoms which closely resemble modern day Parkinson's disease. The key observed symptoms were Kampa(tremor), Sthambha(rigidity), Chestasanga(slowness of movement), Vak Vikriti(speech disorder), Avanamana(Flexion Posture), Kshinamati (Dementia), Smritihani (Loss Of Memory) and Vivandha (Constipation).

PD is also defined in ancient Chinese medical sources. The first Chinese medical book, *Yellow Emperor's Internal Classic* describes that tremors and stiffness arise from Yin Yang imbalance. Various Chinese physicians like Zhang Zhonjing, Zhong Ziha and Sun Simiao have described Parkinson's disease-like symptoms. Another famous Chinese physician of the Ming Dynasty, Wang Kentang described the use of an anti-tremor pill in his book *"Ru Men Shi Qin"*. [2]

French neurologist Jean-Martin Charcot further refined Parkinson's description, differentiating it from other disorders and coining the term "Parkinsonism."

Meanwhile, advances in neuropathology revealed the tell-tale hallmarks of the disease - the loss of dopamine-producing cells in the brain's substantia nigra. The 20th century became a battlefield against Parkinson's disease with emerging technologies and treatments for curing the disease. However, the exact cure was elusive yet the progress grew louder with every passing year.

While Parkinson's whispers in the shadows, the human spirit dances a defiant waltz. Icons like Muhammad Ali and Michael J. Fox have turned their platforms into stages for awareness and hope. Their stories urge us to listen beyond the tremors and celebrate the quiet victories.

Parkinson's isn't just a chronicle of the past; it's a springboard for the future. As we turn the page, let's carry the spirit of resilience, honoring past struggles and paving the way for a future where movement's melody rings loud and clear.

Chapter 2- Unveiling the whispers within: Recognizing the symptoms of Parkinson's disease

Parkinson's disease evokes images of trembling hands and shuffling gait but this insidious melody plays a far more complex symphony, often starting with subtle notes that can mimic the ageing process itself. The patient may look good even when they don't feel good.

The symptoms of the disease can be motor and non-motor symptoms which can be classified as Early symptoms and Late symptoms.

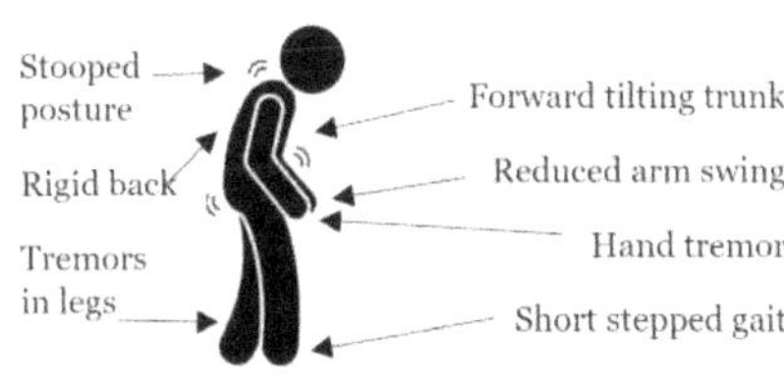

Visual symptoms of Parkinson's

A person in the later stages of Parkinson's disease can be recognized with a stooped posture and a staggering gait.

The motor symptoms of Parkinson's include tremors, rigidity, spasticity, bradykinesia and loss of balance; whereas, the non-motor symptoms include depression, diarrhea, constipation, urinary urgency, loss of sense of smell, dream enactment behavior, depression and anxiety.

Early Stage Symptoms

Hoehn & Yahr defined 5 stages of Parkinson's Disease:

Stage 1:

In the early stages of the condition, symptoms are often subtle and minimally disruptive to a person's daily routine.

Tremors at rest: The disease begins with slight shaking of the limbs, which can also be felt in other parts of the body.

Bradykinesia: The person's gait becomes unsteady and slow.

Stage 2:

The disease progresses, leading to a worsening of tremors. The symptoms now affect both sides of the body or the core (neck and trunk). Difficulty walking and impaired posture become more noticeable.

Rigidity: The limbs become stiff leading to reduction in arm and leg movement.

Flexed posture: The person's posture curves forward. As the disease progresses, the patient's posture becomes permanently stooped, their muscles become even weaker, and they can barely support themselves.

Violent tremors: As the condition progresses, tremors escalate in intensity, transforming into uncontrollable shakes that impede daily life. Walking becomes extremely difficult, as each step requires immense effort to lift legs even a few centimeters. Feeding oneself transforms into a battle, demanding every ounce of focus to guide trembling hands towards the mouth. Handwriting deteriorates, shrinking into a spidery scrawl that defies comprehension.

They have less control over their movements. Daily activities like holding a pen or a spoon become a task. The muscles in the limbs that do not move much waste away and become weak. While independent living remains possible, daily tasks become increasingly challenging and time-consuming.

Mid-stage Symptoms

Stage 3:

Loss of postural reflexes: It leads to the loss of balance. The patient's difficulty in moving their body forces them to walk on their toes and the forepart of their feet only. To prevent falling, they take quicker and shorter steps, which gives the impression that they are running unwillingly. This increases the risk of falling.

More frequent falls: The risk of falling becomes more significant at this stage.

Worsening motor symptoms: Tremor, rigidity, and slowness of movement will continue to progress.

Limited daily activities: While independence is still possible, some daily tasks may become more challenging.

Mild to moderate disability: Individuals may experience limitations in their daily lives but can still manage most activities.

Later Stage Symptoms

Stage 4:

Severe symptoms: Tremor, rigidity, slowness of movement, and other symptoms are at their most pronounced.

Limited mobility: While still able to walk and stand independently for short periods, using a cane or walker becomes necessary for safety and increased support.

Extensive care needs: Daily activities like bathing, dressing, and eating require significant assistance.

Inability to live independently: Living alone becomes unsafe, and full-time care is typically required.

Stage 5:

The most advanced stage of Parkinson's disease is marked by severe limitations. Leg stiffness can become so pronounced that standing or walking independently is no longer possible. Individuals in this stage may be bedridden or require a wheelchair for mobility, and rely on constant assistance for all daily activities.

Freezing phenomenon: During a freeze response, someone might feel rooted to the spot, unable to move even a muscle. They might be stuck in their chair, as if glued down. Even talking could become a struggle.

Non-motor symptoms:

As the disease advances, the patient starts experiencing non-motor symptoms.

- **Sleep disorders**-Parkinson's disease can severely disrupt sleep. Patients may experience involuntary muscle contractions during sleep, which can wake them up. This makes them impatient and they are frustrated. Some patients may even shout or cry out in their sleep. Many people with Parkinson's also have **rapid eye movement sleep behaviour disorder (RBD)**. In this the patient may act of their dream. The patient may show symptoms like jumping from the bed, kicking as well as punching.

- **Restless leg syndrome (RLS)** is another common sleep disorder that can affect people with Parkinson's. RLS is characterized by an urge to move the legs, and it can make it difficult to fall asleep or stay asleep.

- **Autonomic Nervous System failure:** Symptoms of autonomic failure in patients with Parkinson's disease include constipation, urinary incontinence, orthostatic or postprandial light-headedness, and heat or cold intolerance, and signs include decreased bowel sounds and orthostatic hypotension. (Goldstein, 2014)

- **Depression and loss of appetite:** The patient with Parkinson's feels depressed and eats less. Another reason is that they have difficulty in swallowing food as their tongue, pharynx, and other parts of the mouth are impaired.

  They also have difficulty retaining the food in their mouth until it is chewed. Therefore, the saliva fails to be directed to the back of the throat, and it instead drains from the mouth, mixed with particles of food that the patient is no longer able to clear from their mouth.

  Since they eat insufficient food, it makes their bowels irregular and torpid. They require stimulating medication or external aid to expel the feces.

- **Other disabilities:** They find it hard to lift their hands. Chores like putting on or removing clothes become extremely difficult. Additionally, the patient's speech becomes barely intelligible. The advanced stages involve substantial disability, deformity in spine column and peripheral joints generally requiring a wheelchair for movement. The patient might finally become bedbound.

Medication-induced Symptoms

Dyskinesia:

It is the side-effect of Levadopa, the best drug to treat Parkinsonism. Progression of the disease can lead to 'wearing off' episodes of Levodopa, which can become significantly more debilitating than the initial symptoms.

It can be described as involuntary, unpredictable, twisting movement that can affect the face, arms, legs, or trunk. It can be fluid and dance-like, but it can also be rapid, jerky, or slow and sustained.

Psychosis:

Psychosis is a mental health condition that causes people to lose touch with reality. This can manifest as hallucinations, delusions, or disorganized thinking.

Hallucinations are sensory experiences that occur in the absence of an external stimulus. For example, someone with hallucinations might hear voices or see things that are not there.

Delusions are false beliefs that are not shared by others. For example, someone with delusions might believe that they are being followed or that their thoughts are being controlled by someone else.

Obsessive compulsive behaviors:

Dopamine[7] activates the reward center of the brain thereby leading to impulse control problems. Some patients may develop obsessive compulsive[8] behavior towards gambling, sex, and shopping.

Sleep attacks:

Sleep attacks are sudden, uncontrollable episodes of sleep that can occur in people with Parkinson's disease. These disorders get enhanced and the patients sleep at any time without any warning. They can range from brief moments to minutes or

---

[7] Some people who have Parkinson's disease (PD) will develop compulsive behaviours while receiving dopamine-replacement therapy. Parkinson's Foundation.

[8] Hamilton. (2014). *The Parkinson's you don't see- Cognitive and non-motor symptoms.* Davis Phinney Foundation for Parkinson's.

even hours. They can occur at any time but are more common during the late afternoons and early evenings.

Non-visual symptoms

There are various non-visual symptoms of Parkinson's that are more troublesome than the disease itself. They comprise various cognitive problems like the difficulty in problem solving, planning, organizing, decision making, and thinking. The patients may find it hard to retrieve words and may remain stuck on a single topic. They also develop anxiety, depression, sleep disturbance, constipation, difficulty with temperature regulation. Some patients may also lose their sense of smell much before the motor symptoms start to appear.

Memory problems:

The memory problems associated with Parkinson's are different from those seen in Alzheimer's disease. In Alzheimer's, there is a steady decline in memory, while in Parkinson's, the memory problems can fluctuate throughout the day or week.

People with Parkinson's may find it difficult to keep up with their thoughts, and they may experience waves of confusion. They may also feel confident at one moment and lost the next. Their minds may feel hazy, and they may have trouble concentrating.

Social Communication Challenges in Parkinson's Disease

Patients with Parkinson's disease may find it difficult to socialize well with others. Their face looks like a blank canvas with blurred thoughts. It is generally characterized by the following:

Facial masking

People with Parkinson's disease often have difficulty displaying facial expressions, a symptom known as facial masking. This is due to the slowness of movement (bradykinesia) of the muscles used for facial expressions. Facial masking can occur on both sides of the face, even though Parkinson's disease typically affects one side of the body more than the other.

It is important to note that people with Parkinson's disease who have facial masking do not experience a decrease in their ability to feel emotions. They simply cannot show their emotions on their faces. This can be frustrating for people with Parkinson's, as it can make it difficult to communicate with others and can lead to social isolation.

Facial masking can make it difficult for people with Parkinson's Disease to smile, frown, or show other facial expressions.

Facial masking can make people with Parkinson's disease appear indifferent or emotionless even when they are feeling strong emotions.

Facial masking can make it difficult for people with the disease to communicate effectively with others and can lead to social isolation.

There is no cure for facial masking in Parkinson's disease, but there are treatments that can help to improve it. These treatments include medication, physical therapy, and speech therapy.

People with Parkinson's disease are often unable to smile naturally, which can have a significant impact on their social interactions. Parkinson's disease can affect the muscles used for smiling, making it difficult to raise the corners of the mouth and eyes. This can result in smiles that appear forced or fake, which can lead others to perceive the person with the disease as being cold or withdrawn.

A study by Simons et al. found that only 73% of Parkinson's disease patients smiled when they were given a surprise gift, compared to 84% of healthy controls. Of the Parkinson's disease patients who did smile, only 36% produced a genuine smile, known as a Duchenne smile. Duchenne smiles involve the contraction of muscles around the eyes, as well as the mouth. Non-Duchenne smiles, on the other hand, do not involve the contraction of the muscles around the eyes.

Duchenne smiles are considered to be more genuine and sincerer than non-Duchenne smiles. They also elicit more positive emotions in others, such as empathy and pleasure. This is why the loss of the ability to produce Duchenne smiles can have negative social consequences for people with Parkinson's disease. They may be avoided or excluded by others, which can make it difficult to maintain relationships.

Emotional recognition problem

People with Parkinson's disease may have difficulty recognizing the emotions of others. Some studies have found that people with Parkinson's disease have difficulty recognizing emotions in general, while others have found that they have difficulty recognizing specific emotions, such as anger or sadness. Still other studies have found no difference in emotion recognition ability between people with Parkinson's disease and healthy controls.

The inconsistent findings in the research are likely due to a number of factors, including the variability of the methods used to assess emotion recognition and the heterogeneity of the Parkinson's disease patient population. More research is needed to better understand the nature of potential deficits in emotion recognition among people with Parkinson's disease.

Dysarthria

Parkinson's disease can cause speech to become abnormal and monotonous, a condition known as dysarthria.

Dysarthria is characterized by a loss of the musical quality of speech, which conveys emotion and meaning. People with the disease who have dysarthria may speak in a slow, halting manner with a harsh voice and inappropriate pauses.

Dysarthria may only occur during spontaneous speech, such as when talking with friends or family. It may not occur when singing or reading aloud.

The effect of dopaminergic medication on dysarthria in Parkinson's disease is not fully understood. Some studies have found that levodopa, a common medication for Parkinson's Disease, can improve some aspects of speech, such as vowel articulation. However, other studies have found that levodopa has little effect on speech intelligibility or prosody.

Despite the lack of clear evidence, dysarthria can be a distressing and isolating condition for people with the disease. This is because it can make it difficult to communicate with others and can lead to social withdrawal.

Prosody identification deficit

People with Parkinson's disease may have difficulty recognizing the emotional prosody of others' speech, even though they can still produce expressive speech. Emotional prosody is the use of pitch, intonation, and rhythm to convey emotion. People with the disease may have difficulty identifying specific negative emotions, such as fear, anger, and disgust, as well as the overall emotional tone of a person's speech.

The inconsistent findings in this area are likely due to a number of factors, including methodological differences and sample variability. More research is needed to clarify the effect of dopaminergic therapy on prosody recognition in Parkinson's disease.

Thus, it can be concluded that the symptoms of Parkinson's disease can vary widely from person to person and can also change over time. While the classic symptoms of the disease remain most prevalent and obvious, the non-motor symptoms are as troublesome as them.

When I start pouring [cereal], I don't know what's going to happen. The next thing I know, I'm spraying All-Bran all over the kitchen.

MICHAEL J. FOX

Chapter 3: Deciphering the Code: A Systematic Exploration of the Causative Factors for Parkinson's disease

The cause of Parkinson's disease is a mystery that has vexed scientists for centuries. Early research suggested that the disease was caused by a genetic mutation, as it often ran in families. However, this theory was challenged by the discovery that many people with Parkinson's disease had no family history of the disease.

In recent years, scientists have begun to explore the possibility that Parkinson's disease is caused by a combination of genetic and environmental factors. This theory is supported by the fact that people with certain genetic mutations are more likely to develop Parkinson's disease, and that environmental factors such as exposure to pesticides and herbicides can also increase the risk of the disease.

The discovery that Parkinson's disease can occur in young people is also a puzzle. The disease is typically diagnosed in people over the age of 60, but there have been cases of people as young as 20 developing the disease. This suggests that there may be other factors that contribute to the development of the disease, such as exposure to toxins or infections.

The mystery of Parkinson's disease is still far from being solved. However, the research that has been conducted so far has provided valuable insights into the possible causes of the disease. This research is leading to the development of new treatments and prevention strategies, and it is giving hope to the millions of people who are affected by Parkinson's disease. This finding prompted researchers to explore alternative explanations for the cause of Parkinson's disease.

The first documentation of Parkinson's disease in 1817 coincided with the Industrial Revolution, a time when coal was the primary fuel source and released countless toxins into the environment. This has led to the question of whether Parkinson's disease is caused by man-made toxins, such as neurotoxic metals like lead and mercury.

The Industrial Revolution was a period of rapid economic and technological growth, but it also came with a significant cost to human health. The burning of coal released harmful pollutants into the air, water, and soil. These pollutants can damage the nervous system, and they have been linked to a number of health problems, including Parkinson's disease.

In recent years, there has been growing evidence that exposure to environmental toxins can increase the risk of developing Parkinson's disease. For example, a study of people living in areas with high levels of air pollution found that they were more likely to develop Parkinson's disease than those living in areas with lower levels of pollution.

While the exact role of environmental toxins in the development of Parkinson's disease is still not fully understood, the evidence suggests that they may play a significant role.

In 1983, Dr. J. William Langston, a renowned neurologist at Stanford University, made a startling discovery. He found that a group of heroin addicts in California were developing Parkinson's-like symptoms. These addicts had injected a synthetic opioid called MPTP, which had properties similar to those of heroin. However, MPTP also had a devastating side effect: it could cause instant Parkinson's disease, affecting the exact same area of the brain.

Langston's discovery was a major breakthrough in the understanding of Parkinson's disease. It showed that the disease could be caused by a toxin, and it led to the development of new animal models of Parkinson's disease. These models have been invaluable in research, and they have helped to identify new targets for drug development.

The discovery of MPTP, a toxin that can cause Parkinson's-like symptoms, sparked a flurry of research into the environmental causes of the disease. However, no single environmental factor has been definitively linked to Parkinson's disease, although some studies have suggested that exposure to pesticides may increase the risk of developing the disease by as much as 70%.

Dr. J. William Langston, who first identified MPTP as a cause of Parkinson's, has suggested that the disease may be caused by a combination of different factors, including genetics, environmental exposure, and age. While the exact cause of Parkinson's remains unknown, the discovery of MPTP has helped to shed light on the disease and has led to the development of new animal models that can be used to study the disease and test potential treatments.

Genetics of Parkinson's disease

Across our 23 pairs of chromosomes, researchers have pinpointed 28 regions likely linked to Parkinson's disease. However, only six of these regions hold genes with confirmed mutations that directly cause a specific form of Parkinson's disease known as monogenic Parkinson's disease, where a single faulty gene triggers the disease. Even combining these six genes' mutations explains only a small fraction of Parkinson's disease cases (3-5% of sporadic occurrences).

Idiopathic disease

Until a definitive cause of Parkinson's is identified, the disease will remain an idiopathic disease, meaning that it has no known cause.

While many environmental toxins have been suspected of triggering Parkinson's disease, the evidence remains murky. [9]

Some studies hint at a link between Parkinson's disease and occupational exposure to chemicals, particularly in agriculture with pesticides and heavy metals. However, other professions like electricians, exposed to low-frequency magnetic fields, or those working with diesel fumes and solvents, haven't shown such connections.

The relationship between rural living and Parkinson's disease has been a hot debate. Some studies find no association, even suggesting an urban edge to the disease. Others in densely populated cities link the risk of Parkinson's disease to industrial air pollution, heavy metals, and traffic emissions. Yet, other studies find no geographical trend, while some associate rural exposure with higher risk. This could be partly due to a larger aging population in rural areas.

Therefore, the impact of the environment on Parkinson's disease is complex and requires

---

[9] (Nicole Ball, 2019). *Parkinson's Disease and the Environment,* NIH

further investigation. While occupational exposure to certain chemicals might play a role, the picture isn't clear-cut across different professions and locations.

Deciphering this environmental puzzle necessitates more extensive research and a nuanced understanding of factors like age distribution across various settings.

Chapter 4 -The Quest for a Cure: The Current Landscape of Parkinson's Disease Research

"The cures we want aren't going to fall from the sky. We have to get ladders, and climb up to get them."

-MICHAEL J. FOX

In 1817, Dr. James Parkinson first described the neurogenetic disease that would later bear his name.

In the mid-19th century, French neurologist Martin Charcot distinguished Parkinson's from other tremulous disorders and identified several atypical variants of the disease, which he grouped under the Parkinsonism-plus syndrome.

Following the 1916-17 influenza epidemic, a new and more common disorder emerged, known as post-encephalic parkinsonism. This condition was believed to be caused by a viral illness that triggered the degeneration of nerve cells in the substantia nigra. However, the epidemic ended and the patients died, and the condition disappeared with them.

The first established treatment for Parkinson's disease was developed in 1972 by Dr. Ordenstein, who advocated the use of belladonna alkaloids.

After a series of unsuccessful research, J M Charcot designed a vibratory chair to treat patients, observing that they felt more comfortable and slept better as a result.

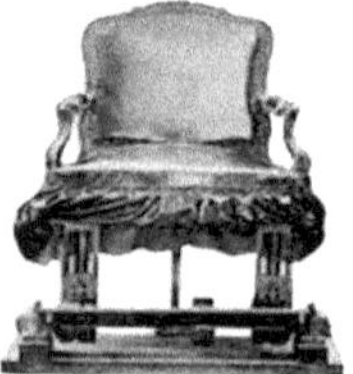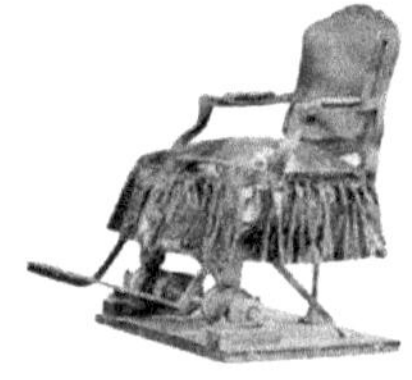

"Vibration chair" by Jean Martin Charcot

However, Charcot died before doing further comprehensive studies using his device.

Charcot even advocated that the patients of Parkinson's were not weak and thus calling the disease as "palsy" was not justified and thus the disease should be called Parkinson's disease".

WR Growers, who was a British contemporary of Charcot used hyoscyamine, *ob*[10] and *opium* in

---

[10] Goetz, Christopher. *The History of Parkinson's Disease: Early Clinical Descriptions and Neurological Therapies*, NIH

combination. They are known to increase the dopamine concentration in the blood.[11]

In the early 20th century, the treatment of Parkinson's disease was limited to supportive physical therapy and management of symptoms. This included treating hypersalivation, scaly skin patches, and infections.

In 1910, dopamine was first synthesized by G. Barger and J. Ewens. The following year, Casimir Funk synthesized dopa, the precursor to dopamine. In 1913, Marcus Guggenheim isolated dopa from the broad bean (*Vicia faba*) plant. However, at the time, dopa was thought to be a toxin with no biological use.

In 1960, Swedish pharmacologist Arvid Carlsson presented a paper at the Ciba Foundation Symposium on Adrenergic Mechanism in London, proposing that dopamine was a neurotransmitter and implicated it with Parkinson's disease. His concepts were rejected by the scientific community.

However, in 1961, Australian scientist Oleh Hornykeiwicz decided to look at the levels of dopamine in the post-mortem brains of patients with Parkinson's disease. He concluded that the symptoms of Parkinson's disease could be due to the lack of dopamine.

In the same year, he joined hands with neurologist Walter Birkmayer. They achieved

---

[11] Oleson, Eric, (2012). *A Brain on Cannabinoids: The Role of Dopamine Release in Reward Seeking*. NIH

temporary yet miraculous transformations by the use of Levodopa (precursor of dopamine) in the patients with Parkinson's disease.

In 1968, oral trials of Levodopa began. The drug was approved by the US Food and Drug Administration in 1970.

Since then it has become the widely used dopamine replacement agent to reduce classic motor symptoms like slowness of movement (bradykinesia), and rigidity in Parkinson's disease.

Problems with Levodopa

Levodopa started to be used widely in the treatment of Parkinson's. Even though it brought some relief to the patients, it also led to various problematic side effects.

Common side effects:

Nausea, sleepiness, dizziness, and headaches. These can often be managed by starting with a low dose and increasing gradually.

More serious side effects:

Hallucinations[12], vision problems cognitive impairment, excessive motor fluctuations i.e.

---

[12] Stoker TB, Greenland JC. (2018). *Parkinson's Disease: Pathogenesis and Clinical Aspects*. NIH

frequent movement of limbs, dyskinesia, delusions, agitation, and psychosis. These are more likely in older patients.

Motor fluctuations: This is when the medication wears off before the next dose, leading to symptoms returning.

Other drugs used to treat Parkinson's Disease

Carbidopa with levodopa: When carbidopa is taken along with levodopa it inhibits peripheral metabolism of levodopa i.e. the breakdown of levodopa before it reaches the brain. This helps the patients take lower doses of levodopa which causes less vomiting and nausea. Carbidopa alone has no benefits. One such combination is sold by the brand name: Sinemet.

Dopamine agonists: Dopamine agonist drugs act like imposters, fooling your brain into believing they're real dopamine. This helps mimic dopamine's natural effects and ease the symptoms. These are usually prescribed in the early stages of the disease. The various agonists are Pramipexole, Ropinirole, Rotigotine Transdermal Patch and Apomorphine. [13]

---

[13] S Bunten. (2006) *Rotigotine transdermal system: a short review.* NIH

Benefits:

- Delay dopamine treatment.
- Lower the risk of dyskinesia, dystonia and motor fluctuations as compared to Levodopa.
- Help in reducing the dose of Levodopa.
- Help in treating restless leg syndrome.

Side effects: While slightly less effective than Levodopa, dopamine agonists come with more potential side effects like nausea, vomiting, dry mouth, constipation, fainting, drowsiness, leg swelling, hallucinations, sleepiness and even uncontrollable urges to gamble, eat, or shop.

MAO-B inhibitors (rasagiline, selegiline, safinamide):

A brain enzyme called MAO-B naturally breaks down dopamine, a key chemical for movement. MAO-B inhibitors block this enzyme, allowing more dopamine to work in the brain. This can slightly improve the symptoms of Parkinson's disease, especially those related to movement.[14]

MAO-B inhibitors, like Eldepryl, Emsam, Zelapar (selegiline), Azilect (rasagiline), and Xadago (safinamide), can help manage Parkinson's disease symptoms, especially the "wearing off" effect when Levodopa wears out. Some, like

---

[14] Yu-Yan Tan, Peter Jenner, and Sheng-Di Chen. (2022). *Monoamine Oxidase-B Inhibitors for the Treatment of Parkinson's Disease: Past, Present, and Future.* NIH

selegiline and rasagiline, can even be used alone in the early stages of the disease.

Side effects: While MAO-B inhibitors can help with Parkinson's, they come with potential side effects like indigestion, nausea, headaches, and sleep problems.

In older adults with the disease, confusion caused by selegiline can be a concern. It's important to note that combining these medications with antidepressants carries a very rare but serious risk called serotonin syndrome.[15]

COMT Inhibitors: These medications work by blocking an enzyme called COMT (catechol-o-methyl-transferase), which normally breaks down a drug called Levodopa outside the brain. This prevents Levodopa from being destroyed before it reaches the brain, allowing more to enter and improve symptoms.[16]

It includes drugs like Tasmar (tolcapone), Comtan (entacapone), and Ongentys (opicapone) that help boost the effectiveness of levodopa, extending its duration and improving its impact on Parkinson's symptoms.

Side effects:

Taking COMT inhibitors comes with potential side effects like uncontrollable movements

---

[15] Chou KL. (2023) *Serotonin syndrome is a life-threatening condition that occurs due to the overactivity of serotonin in the brain.* PARKINSON DISEASE OVERVIEW
[16] Rivest, J. *COMT inhibitors in Parkinson's disease.* NIH

(dyskinesia), hallucinations, confusion, nausea, diarrhoea, orange urine, and dizziness upon standing.

Amantadine: Amantadine helps ease some Parkinson's symptoms, possibly by boosting dopamine levels in the brain.

In the early stages, it can improve slow movements and stiffness. Later on, it can be combined with other drugs like Sinemet® to reduce involuntary movements caused by those medications.[17]

Side effects:

Taking amantadine can come with side effects like seeing things that aren't there (hallucinations), feeling confused, developing purple skin patches (livedo reticularis) and swelling in ankles.

Anticholinergics: In Parkinson's disease, a brain chemical called acetylcholine becomes overactive, causing tremors. Anticholinergic drugs work by blocking this chemical, calming the overactive area and reducing tremors.[18]

The medication includes trihexyphenidyl, benztropine, orphenadrine, procyclidine, and biperiden. They are considered effective in treating symptoms.

---

[17] Bailey, EV. *The mechanism of action of amantadine in Parkinsonism: a review.* NIH

[18] Chou KL. (2023). PARKINSON DISEASE OVERVIEW

Side Effects:

Taking anticholinergic medications for Parkinson's can bring relief, but also potential side effects like dry mouth, blurry vision, constipation, and trouble with digestion or urination. They can also affect sweating and heart rate. In some cases, memory, confusion, and even hallucinations might occur.

Right time to start PD medication

There isn't a single "right time" to begin Parkinson's medication for everyone. The decision is a collaborative effort between the patient and the doctor, considering the impact of symptoms on daily life.

Typically, medication isn't started immediately after diagnosis, particularly if symptoms are mild and manageable.

But since tremors, stiffness, or slowness of movement can significantly affect the ability to work, socialize, or perform daily activities, medication can be a valuable tool to improve the quality of life and therefore it is advisable to start the medication as soon as the symptoms start appearing.

Ultimately, the best approach is to discuss your specific situation with the doctor to determine the optimal time to initiate Parkinson's medication.

Chapter 5- The Patient Odyssey: Analyzing the Unique Journeys

The enigma of Parkinson's disease lies in its ability to touch so many lives in such disparate ways. The symptoms of the disease can manifest themselves in a variety of ways, and the rate of progression can vary greatly from person to person. As a result, many people are not diagnosed until the disease is in its later stages.

Case 1: 74-year-old musician dropped her Sitar

On a balmy morning at Versova Beach, 74-year-old Urmi decided to recapture her youth. She returned to her cozy sea-facing apartment and retrieved her most cherished possession: her Sitar.

Urmi tried to lift the heavy musical instrument, but her hands jerked and she dropped it. The instrument was not damaged, but a few strings were broken. This was the first time that Urmi realized she had a pressing problem to deal with.

The incidents of falling, bumping into objects, and dropping things were getting frequent.

"I remember breaking my shoulder bone by falling off the stairs. It took a lot of time to heal. But my Sitar made me reconsider my situation seriously", recalls Urmi.

Urmi lives with her loving son in the suburbs of Mumbai. Music and dance were her life. But her life has turned sedentary for a very long time. The incident further enhanced her depression. The medicines she took to treat depression were causing sleepiness and weight gain that further added to lethargy. The kaleidoscope of her life has lost its colors. Many months passed by when one fine day Urmi decided to change things.

"I was losing control over my life", she complained.

On diagnosis, it was confirmed that she suffered from Parkinson's disease. She knew about the disease as her sister-in-law was suffering from the same. She was prescribed medication for it.

"I hated the medicines I took for depression, but not as much as I hate the Parkinson's medicines", stated Urmi.

The drugs for depression made her sleep as they relax the body and the mind. However, the medicines for Parkinson's had their side effects which she totally disliked. She suffered from hallucinations and so she asked her neurologist to change her medication.

Her gait was changing and her posture was stooping. There was no visual shaking of limbs but they had stiffness. Thus, a physiotherapist was appointed for her.

On a warm summer morning, Urmi's son burst into the house with the joyous news of a new addition to the family. Urmi was beside herself with excitement. She had always dreamed of being a grandmother, and now her dream was coming true.

In her eagerness to hold the baby in her arms, Urmi began exercising. She cooperated with her physical therapist more and focused more on doing things herself.

She started with small steps, afraid of falling. But as she continued to exercise, her fear of falling abated and she was filled with the desire to move forward.

To help her achieve her fitness goals, Urmi joined a dance class. She had always loved Kathak, a graceful and expressive form of Indian dance. At first, it was difficult. Urmi's body didn't move the way it used to. She had tremors and stiffness. But she kept practicing, and gradually, she started to improve.

The more she danced, the better she felt. The exercise helped to control her symptoms, and it also gave her a sense of joy and purpose. She started to feel like herself again.

Urmi continued to dance. She even started teaching dance to other people with Parkinson's disease. Her next goal was to start her Sitar lessons. It was difficult to move her fingers on the instrument swiftly but she managed to practice.

Her faith in herself and the desire to live fully in touch with reality made her live better with the disease.

She even began singing. It helped in improving her speech as well as her swallowing problem.

She became an example of courage that can change lives. She showed everyone it is possible to live a full and active life with the disease even at a later age.

Case 2: 84-year-old Sarika Mitra diagnosed with depression

Sarika Mitra was a professor of eminence at a government college, where she had served for 35 illustrious years. She lived a contented single life, caring for her aging parents. Her social circle was small but close-knit; her friends considered her family, and her life was joyful. As her retirement drew nearer, she decided to build a house in her hometown.

Fate had other plans for her. As her active life vanished after her retirement, she found herself sinking into the depths of depression.

She took antidepressant pills for 2 years. She had been experiencing a decline in her social circle and physical mobility. Within the next 6 months there were a series of episodes of objects falling from her hands. Her family initially ignored these symptoms. But, in the next 1 month, the shaking of her limbs was considerably visible that eventually led them to seek medical attention. Finally, the disease was diagnosed as Parkinson's disease.

"I haven't heard the name of this disease before", stated Sarika's sister, Alpana.

As the disease progressed, Sarika's depression deepened. Her symptoms seemed insurmountable. The changes in her eating habits led to a dramatic weight loss. The medications were changed countless times in an effort to find the right dosage.

Adding to that, there were innumerable personality changes that were difficult to decipher.

"We made every effort to keep her happy and engaged in activities she enjoyed, but she seemed indifferent to everything. She would often become fixated on a single task, such as repeatedly washing her hands for hours at the sink. We would ask her to stop and go to her room, but she would refuse to listen. It was difficult to force her to do anything at that point, and it was a challenging task to manage her", stated her brother, Shaunak.

"We could find her standing anywhere at any time during the day or at night. It was scary at times", added Aunindyo, her nephew.

"Her legs started swelling due to prolonged standing throughout the day", said Alpana.

Those were the initial years of her treatment when the effects of medication were observed. The fluctuating levels of dopamine in blood were leading to certain changes.

"We didn't know that it could be because of the medicine, till the doctor changed it. We thought that the medicine was effective as the shaking of her limbs had ceased." Alpana added.

The shaking had stopped, but the medication was causing different effects on the brain. The doctor changed the medication as well as the dose.

"We changed the medication. But it was required otherwise the symptoms would resurface again", said the neurologist.

"She would become fixated on different tasks at different times. She might stand in one place for hours, or she might make repetitive, annoying sounds. Her behavior was unpredictable.", said Alpana.

The doctors continued with the medication. Most of the time it worked fine but at times there were side effects that became difficult to manage.

The patient visited the physiotherapist regularly in an attempt to improve her mobility, but her progress was limited due to her inflexible attitude and refusal to cooperate. Over time, she became completely immobile, and her feet became increasingly twisted and rigid, despite the physiotherapist's best efforts.

"Her knees were stiff and unyielding, not only from physical limitations, but also from mental anguish. Her lower body was becoming increasingly rigid, and physical activity was essential to her recovery. In contrast, her forelimbs remained relatively supple", said the physiotherapist.

"Once a vivacious conversationalist, she has become subdued over the years. She speaks less now, and I sometimes wonder if she is even following our conversations", added Alpana.

"Her speech was becoming increasingly slurred and unintelligible. A speech therapist was recommended, but her depression was making it difficult for her to recover", said Shaunak.

The patient's declining condition had plunged her into a deep depression, but there were still moments when she could forget her troubles and act like her old self.

"We started counting the number of days when she would be totally normal. There were no signs of depression or Parkinson's disease, as if it never existed. She would eat, laugh and joke. We celebrate her normal days", stated Alpana.

"During the day, we kept her busy with people and music to distract her from her troubles. However, the most difficult part was the night. She had trouble sleeping and often experienced hallucinations. She would see thieves, robberies, and sick people, and we believed her until she started talking to imaginary people. This usually happened at night, and she would sleep for the entire day after a night of intense hallucinations", stated Aunindyo.

The doctor advised the physical therapy sessions to be increased. The doses and medication were altered periodically.

"There was a time when she completely gave up on walking. We knew it was not a good sign", told Alpana.

"We knew that walking was one important aspect. Something was required to be done to motivate her", added Shaunak.

The family tried everything they could to get their loved one to walk again, but their efforts were in vain. They consulted a doctor, who altered the dose of her medication. Surprisingly, this worked, and the patient began to talk normally again. She also started walking subconsciously. The family stopped asking her to walk or stand, and instead pretended that she could. To their surprise, she started to try to walk and stand on her own. However, her feet couldn't cooperate and there were risks of falling.

The patient's condition fluctuated daily and weekly. She was better in the summer months than in the winter months, and during the day than at night. She also became more susceptible to cold weather, and needed more protection not only during the winter months but also in the summer months. There were days when her chest would get so congested that she needed to use a nebulizer twice a day.

One night, while the patient was being fed, she started coughing. The family member patting her back tried to stop the coughing, but her face turned red. She was choking. They knew it was an emergency. The patient was rushed to the hospital emergency room, where it was discovered that food had gotten stuck in her trachea/windpipe, causing her to choke. Her oxygen levels dropped to 85%.

"Her oxygen was dangerously low," said the emergency room doctor. The patient was kept in the hospital for monitoring.

Some years passed in making things better and then worse. The ups and downs continued for a much longer time when after 3 years, the patient gave up.

"It became difficult to make her stand anymore. And we knew we couldn't force. Dystonia was clearly visible. Her toes started curling inwards and the muscles of the calf tightened."

The journey so far was just the tip of the iceberg, a mere prelude to the war that lay ahead, a battle tougher than the family had ever imagined.

The patient was bedridden.

"We knew that she would require more care, but we were prepared", said Alpana.

Firstly, to prevent any bed sores, the mattress was changed to an air bed.

"We changed her position four to five times a day to prevent bedsores," Alpana added.

Since it was difficult for the patient to go to the bathroom every time, a urine bag was used.

"However, there was a problem with using a catheter. It requires utmost hygiene to prevent urinary tract infections, and it needs to be changed frequently", Shaunak added.

"One night, I heard some voices coming from her room," Shaunak said. "I looked at the monitor, and she looked fine. But there was still something off."

"I woke Shaunak up," Alpana said. "She was making noise. We decided to go check on her."

"She was hallucinating and talking to herself," Shaunak said. "We tried to calm her down and watched her for a while. Then we realized that she had rotated 180 degrees in bed!"

"In the process, she pulled out her catheter and there was urine all over the bed," Alpana said. "She must have struggled hard to change position in bed. She must have been very disturbed."

The doctor was consulted, and he informed them that the medications were making the patient's brain hyperactive. The medications would adjust over time, and the patient would have some good days and some bad days.

Case 3: A 35-year old woman presents with a 1-year history of progressive tremors

It was on her 32nd birthday that Tanvi realized that she was having difficulty in unwrapping her gifts. Her arms were shaking and she had difficulty in holding objects. She faced immense difficulty in getting out of the bed in the morning. Her gait started becoming unsteady.

She had been observing the change in her abilities since a very long time so she decided to consult a doctor.

She was thus, diagnosed with Young Onset Parkinson's disease (YOPD).

The disease was a setback to her. As the disease progressed, it hampered her progress. Daily chores became difficult.

Despite the tremors that rattled her hands and the stiffness that stole her grace, a fire continued to burn brightly within her.

She has decided to live with the disease and work for her betterment. The journey wasn't easy. There were days when the tremors were relentless, stealing her independence. The world, once a vibrant canvas, seemed muted. Yet, Tanvi fought back. She researched, joining online support groups, learning from others with Parkinson's disease. She embraced medication and physical therapy, the controlled movements a daily struggle, a victory nonetheless. She explored yoga, the slow, deliberate movements a soothing balm to her body. Slowly, her life morphed into a beautiful mosaic – acceptance, resilience, and a fierce determination to live life to the fullest, on her own terms.

The disease might have taken away some things, but it couldn't touch the spirit that danced within, reminding her that life, in all its challenges, was still a beautiful adventure waiting to be explored.

"We all have challenges," she says, "but even in the midst of them, there's beauty to be found. And life, my dear, is always worth living."

Discussion on disease progression

The progression of the cases studied can be made in the following manner. Firstly, it can be said that the cases differed in many ways.

Observations:

- The patient did not have any family history of Parkinson's disease.
- The patient had been taking antidepressants for a long time.
- Side effects of the disease started surfacing.
- The patient started showing repetitive behavior.
- The patient dramatically lost weight over the years.
- Dystonia was observed after a few years.
- Patient gives up on walking completely.
- Physical exercise and walking help in managing the symptoms.
- Singing is also beneficial in improving speech.

Inference:

- The use of antidepressants[19] may have precipitated the onset of Parkinson's

---

[19] Alonso, Rodríguez and Logroscino. (2010) *Use of antidepressants and the risk of Parkinson's disease: a prospective study.* NIH

disease in the patient. This is supported by a study approved by the Institutional Review Board at Harvard School of Public Health, which found that initiation of any antidepressant therapy was associated with a significantly increased risk of Parkinson's disease in the two years following treatment.

- During the initial stages some drugs at the existing dosage cause side effects. They are required to be adjusted in the drug regime. The drugs are introduced at low doses which are gradually increased over weeks or months. Therefore, the drugs take some months to develop their full effect.
- The symptoms of Parkinson's disease occur in waves. When the medication suits, then the patient seems to be normal. If time and dosage of medicines is changed, the symptoms may start surfacing.
- People with Parkinson's disease may have weak muscles in their throat, which can make it difficult to swallow food. If food gets stuck in the trachea, it can cause aspiration pneumonia, a serious infection. Aspiration pneumonia can be life-threatening, especially in people with Parkinson's disease.
- Dystonia is a common movement disorder that affects up to 30% of people with Parkinson's disease. It is characterized by involuntary muscle contractions that can

cause the body to twist into unnatural postures. Dystonia is more likely to occur in people with Parkinson's disease who develop the condition before the age of 40 [20] i.e. Young onset PD. It particularly involves lower limbs.

Most Parkinson's patients take levodopa at some point. Long-term use and disease progression can lead to motor complications. Motor fluctuations are changes in how well levodopa works. This can cause Parkinson's symptoms to come and go, or get worse at certain times of day. Dystonia is generally a part of the "off" periods. However, it can also occur during the on periods. The "Off" periods are when Parkinson's symptoms are worse, even though the patient is taking levodopa. They can be caused by a number of factors, including low levels of dopamine in the brain, changes in the dose of levodopa, or other medications.

- The fear of falling takes away the confidence to walk independently. It is enhanced by stiffness and curling of toes.

---

[20] Shetty, Bhaita and Lang. (2019) *Dystonia and Parkinson's disease: What is the relationship?* Neurobiology of Disease

Chapter 6- The Caregiver's Compass: Essential Strategies for Life with Parkinson's

"By the time we realized, our lives had already changed and there was no going back", recalls Tuhina, a Parkinson's caregiver.

The journey with Parkinson's disease is unique for each individual, and so is the role of the care partner. There is no one-size-fits-all definition of caregiving, and what it means may change over time. A person who is a Parkinson's caregiver knows that the role cannot be summed up in one sentence.

Caregiving can be physical, emotional, and spiritual. Responsibilities range from (and are not limited to) helping the patient in performing daily chores like preparing meals, housekeeping, shopping, laundry, managing medications and offering emotional support to full-time monitoring of patients and handling them during a chaotic phase of psychosis. During the advanced stages of the disease, patients require assistance in bathing, grooming, dressing, toileting, getting in and out of the wheelchair, car or shower. They require a cheerleader, a companion and an emotionally available person.

There are millions of people that aid patients of Parkinson's disease all over the world. These caregivers can be categorized into different types such as: the crisis caregivers, working caregivers, spousal caregivers, long-distance caregivers and the sandwich caregivers. Crisis-caregivers are the ones that step-in only after the patient undergoes a critical situation. While the working caregivers are the people who care for the patients while they are also the bread-earners for their families. Spousal caregivers are the ones who take care of their spouses when they get ill. Long distance caregivers are the ones who live at different places but also provide financial, medical and personal care to the patients. Caregivers who are supporting both aging family members and young children at home are called Sandwich caregivers.

Accept the new role

When a loved one is diagnosed with Parkinson's disease, a caregiver is born. Their journey changes as the disease progresses. In the early stages, the patient may not need much care, but as the disease advances, they will require physical, mental, and emotional support. The caregiver's role can be overwhelming if not managed well. Some caregivers lose their sense of self during this process. Embracing the caregiver role shouldn't erase one's identity. Prioritizing self-care strengthens caregiving abilities.

Learn about the disease

A caregiver's journey progresses with the disease of their patients. It becomes utmost important to have a thorough knowledge of the disease in order to participate in various healthcare discussions. It is important to discuss all the symptoms, diagnosis, myths, warning signs, probable emergency situations and fears regarding the medication and treatment.

Make the family understand the disease

It is important for the family members to understand that the disease is more than just a movement disorder. It takes a toll on the mental as well as the emotional health of the patient. It is an ongoing journey in which the patient would need to face realities and make adaptations.

Role of the family

Families play a crucial role in supporting the patient and caregiver throughout their journey. Each family member should contribute to the best of their ability by participating in the caregiving plan, communicating with the patient about their well-being, and researching and providing information about the disease.

Managing time as a Parkinson's caregiver

Managing time as a Parkinson's disease caregiver can be extremely challenging. It is thus important to find ways to take care and prevent burnout. There are certain things that need to be done:

- Create and follow manageable daily and weekly to-do lists. The most important or difficult tasks need to be prioritized.
- Take advantage of technology. There are a number of applications in our phones that can help in managing our tasks such as, medication reminders, fall detectors, remote care monitoring cameras.
- Batch errands to save time and energy.
- Take a small task when it is required to wait somewhere.

- Delegation of tasks needs to be done whenever possible. Unnecessary tasks should be eliminated.
- Short breaks are necessary in case the caregiving becomes overwhelming.
- Overextending in should be avoided in any situation.
- Large tasks should be broken into smaller, and more manageable chunks.
- Establishment and sticking to routines are important.
- It is important to accept that some things are beyond control.
- During the early stages of the disease it is important to encourage the loved ones to work independently. This will help them to maintain their skills and abilities.
- There are many support groups and resources available. These support groups help to connect with other caregivers and get support.

Self-care as a caregiver

Caregiving is demanding and stressful. It is important for the caregiver to take utmost care of themselves to care better for their loved ones. They need to take out some time for themselves every day. They should prioritize their own needs, regular activities and hobbies.

Exercising regularly keeps body and mind fit. They should focus on keeping themselves fit by drinking enough water, taking rest for the desired amount of time, getting regular physical and mental check-ups.

It is important to have limits to prevent any burn out and mental breakdown. Different family members should be asked for help at different times. If they are not available then some paid workers should be involved so as to get the necessary amount of break.

If they face stressful situations then they should consider meditation and yoga. If they find it hard to manage their emotional health then they can also consult a psychologist for help.

> **Prioritizing needs:**
>
> Identification of concerns.
>
> Categorization of concerns according to their priority.
>
> Documentation of action to be taken.
>
> Discussion of ideas with other people.
>
> Formulation of a plan.
>
> Implementation of the plan.
>
> Help should be taken from others.

Role of a Support Team

Caregivers experience a vast and tumultuous array of emotions that can become overwhelming at times. It is therefore imperative to have a support system that addresses emotional and spiritual needs. This could include the healthcare team, family, friends, support groups, or individual support members. People can also seek solace and strength in faith and spiritual activities or practices. It is essential to accept the changes as they occur and to not be ashamed of asking for help, which is a sign of resilience. By prioritizing self-care, caregivers can proactively mitigate the risk of depression and frustration.

Depression in Caregivers

Caregivers are more susceptible to depression and frustration if they lack a robust support system. Depression manifests itself uniquely in each individual, necessitating a tailored approach to treatment. The core symptoms of depression include insomnia, agitation, anorexia, apathy, impaired concentration, suicidal ideation, and feelings of hopelessness and worthlessness.

It can be addressed by:

- Recognizing the signs and symptoms of depression.

- Talking to the doctor or mental health professional. They can assess the symptoms and develop a treatment plan, which may include medication, therapy, or a combination of both.
- Building a support system. This could include family, friends, other caregivers, support groups, or online communities.
- Indulging in activities that are enjoyable, eating healthy foods, getting enough sleep, and exercising regularly can help curb symptoms of depression.
- Identification of stressors and development of coping mechanisms. There are certain things that cause more stress. So, once they are identified, strategies can be developed for coping with them. This may include things like delegating tasks, taking breaks, or finding relaxation techniques.

Chapter 7: Empower Your Body, Empower Your Life: Exercise for Parkinson's Disease Management

Parkinson's disease doesn't have to side-line an active lifestyle. In fact, staying active is a powerful tool to enhance well-being and maximize enjoyment of life. While exercise won't cure the disease, it's crucial for maintaining long-term quality of life.

Physical Exercise

Staying active is a great way to maintain physical balance, stability, strength and flexibility. There are many activities like walking, running, swimming, dancing, pilate, yoga, golf, gardening that keep the body active. Some activities benefit more than the others; however, consistency is more important.

One step should be taken at a time! The activity level should be gradually increased to make exercise sustainable and enjoyable.

Posture should be maintained: The early noticeable changes in a Parkinson's patient can be seen in their posture. The shoulders slump, making it hard for deep breathing and swallowing. Balancing becomes more difficult as the knees and elbows get bent.

Maintaining proper posture: The wall test can be used daily to check for proper shoulder blade and lower back alignment. Flat back position should be for 5 minutes each morning, keeping the head slightly elevated and avoiding any pressure on shoulders or head.

Stretching: Inactivity and poor posture can lead to stiffness. Stretching exercises help maintain joint mobility by gently lengthening muscles. Choosing stretches that are suitable and performing them before and after strengthening exercises is important.

Strengthening exercises: Strengthening exercises involve using muscles repeatedly in a specific way, ensuring they are challenged and grow stronger in a controlled manner.

Back strengthening exercises: Pulling shoulder blades together backwards.

Leg strengthening exercises:

Strengthening of legs while seated: In this one leg is extended at a time. Then it is held for a moment, and then lowered back down. To make it harder, small weights can be added around the ankles.

Importance of exercising:

Boost your physical health: Exercise combats the negative effects of inactivity, develops strength, flexibility, and endurance. This helps in the management of symptoms like:

- Poor posture
- Decreased range of movement
- Muscle weakness
- Fatigue
- Balance issues

Improvement in the mental well-being: Staying active releases endorphins, natural mood boosters that can help fight depression and anxiety, common concerns with Parkinson's disease.

Live a fuller life: Exercise empowers one to stay independent and do the things they love, whether it's walking, dancing, or simply playing with grandkids.

Speech Therapy

Parkinson's disease changes the movement of the muscles of the throat that makes the voice either more breathy or hoarse. Speech becomes garbled lacking the ups and downs of voice. The movement of their mouths becomes tighter and smaller as compared to the normal. They might be trying to shout but the voice perceived by the listener is very feeble. Changes in memory and cognition also affect the speech. Patients find it difficult to communicate with their loved ones.

Activities that help:

- Singing: These exercises can help to improve vocal loudness, clarity, and range. Singing lessons with an expert can lead to complete vocal exercise. Practicing the Sargam (SA, RE, GA, MA, PA, DHA, NI, SA) with full emphasis helps in toning the muscles.
- Vowel pronunciation exercise: This exercise involves pronouncing the vowels (A, E, I, O, U) with full mouth activation and emphasis. Other sounds like "OH", "OO", "MM", "EE" can be produced by pushing from the diaphragm strongly. These should be spoken for at least 15secs.
- Speaking tongue twisters aloud can also enhance the ability to speak clearly. The sound of each word should be exaggerated.
- Breathing exercises like Pranayam have proven benefit in improving breath and supporting speech. Practicing deep breathing, sectional breathing (i.e. Thoracic or chest breathing, abdominal breathing, and clavicular breathing), forceful exhalation from the abdomen in which inhalation is passive (Kapalbbharti pranayam), alternate nostril breathing (inhale from left nostril keeping the right one closed and then close the left nostril and exhale from the right then inhale from

the right nostril keeping the left one closed and then close the right nostril and exhale from the left). This is known as Anulom Vilom Pranayam in Sanskrit.

- Swallowing exercises: These exercises can help to improve the coordination of the muscles involved in swallowing. Swallow more to swallow better.
- Speech therapy is an effective treatment for Parkinson's disease-related speech and swallowing problems. It can help people with Parkinson's disease improve their vocal strength, pitch, articulation, pronunciation, and swallowing. The therapists help their clients to be loud and communicate with projection.

Facial exercises

Facial exercises can help to improve facial muscle strength and tone, reduce facial masking, and improve speech and swallowing in people with Parkinson's disease. These exercises can be done at home or in a clinical setting, and they can be tailored to the individual's needs.

Some examples of facial exercises include:

- Opening and closing mouth.
- Smiling broadly and holding the smile for a few seconds.
- Frowning deeply and hold the frown for a few seconds.
- Wrinkling the forehead as much as possible and then releasing it.
- Pursing lips together to blow a kiss.

- Blinking the eyes rapidly for a few seconds.

It is important to start slow and gradually increase the intensity and duration of the exercises as tolerated. Facial exercises should be done several times a day for the best results.

Hand exercises

Hand exercises can significantly improve hand strength, dexterity, and flexibility in people with Parkinson's disease. These exercises can be done at home or in a clinical setting, and they can be customized to the individual's needs.

Here are some examples of hand exercises:

- Power grip: This exercise helps to strengthen the muscles in the hands and wrists. It is done by making a tight fist and holding it for 5 seconds, and then relaxing. It can be repeated 10 times.
- Finger spread: This exercise helps to improve the flexibility of the fingers. Spreading the fingers as wide as possible and then holding for 5 seconds, then relaxing them. It can also be repeated 10 times.
- Thumb-to-finger tapping: This exercise helps to improve the dexterity of the

fingers. Tap the thumb to each finger, alternating hands. It is repeated 10 times per hand.

- Arm twisting towards each other and then away from each other. It can be repeated 10 times.
- Bending and extending the fingers without closing the fists powerfully and extending the fingers as far and wide as possible. Repetition-10 times.
- Writing: This exercise helps to improve the handwriting. A few lines of text can be written with intermittent breaks. Repetition- 3 times.
- Using tools: This exercise helps to improve the ability to use tools and utensils like picking up a pen, pencil, or other tools. Repetition: 10 times.

It is important to start slow and gradually increase the intensity and duration of the exercises as tolerated. Hand exercises should be done several times a day for the best results.

Laughter Therapy

Laughter is a powerful tool that can have a profound impact on the lives of people with Parkinson's disease. It can reduce stress, improve mood, boost the immune system, relieve pain, and improve sleep.

Laughter yoga is a type of exercise that combines laughter with yoga poses and breathing exercises, can significantly improve the quality of life for people with Parkinson's disease. The study participants reported feeling less depressed, anxious, and stressed after participating in laughter yoga. They also reported having better sleep and more energy.

Motor functions in patients are believed to improve with laughter. The study participants who watched funny videos showed a significant improvement in their walking speed and balance.

While laughter cannot cure Parkinson's disease, it can be a helpful complementary therapy.

Laughter can be incorporated in several ways:

- By joining a laughter yoga class
- Watching funny videos
- Reading funny books or articles
- Spending time with happy people
- Telling jokes or funny stories

Laughter is a gift that we should all embrace. It is a natural way to boost mood, improve health, and connect with others.

Other Therapies:

There are a wide range of complementary therapies that people with Parkinson's disease (PD) may find helpful. These include meditation, massage, acupuncture, music therapy, and art therapy.

Meditation: Meditation is a mind-body practice that involves focusing attention on the present moment. It has been shown to reduce stress and anxiety, which can be helpful for people with Parkinson's disease.

Massage: Massage is a type of physical touch that can help to relax muscles and improve circulation. It can also be helpful for reducing pain and stiffness, which are common symptoms of Parkinson's disease.

Music therapy: Music therapy is the use of music to improve physical, emotional, and cognitive health. It can be helpful for reducing stress, improving mood, and increasing motivation.

Art therapy: Art therapy is the use of art to express emotions and experiences. It can be helpful for reducing stress, improving communication, and increasing self-awareness.

Chapter 8- Two feet, one hope: Winning Back Your Stride   with Parkinson's Disease

"Walking is a man's best medicine."

— Hippocrates

Walking is a forward-moving act that carries us through life. No matter how heavy our souls may be, if we are determined to walk, we will always move forward.

Parkinson's disease (PD) can devastate a person's gait. But slow and steady walking everyday has proven to be beneficial in reducing the symptoms of Parkinson's disease.

Stiff muscles, rigidity, and bradykinesia (slowed movement) make it difficult to take normal steps. In fact, short, shuffling steps are a hallmark of Parkinson's Disease.

Why is walking a problem?

Walking in case of Parkinson's is different from walking in the normal cases. In normal people, walking comes naturally because there is coordination and balance. However, in case of patients with Parkinson's disease, walking becomes a task. It is because the patients with the disease cannot adjust their balance automatically. Thus, every step requires focus and caution.

Common hindrances in walking:

1. Freezing:

    People with Parkinson's find it hard to move their feet forward. Getting up from a chair and start moving ahead is a big task. If they encounter an obstacle in their path or if they have to move through narrow spaces, then they feel that their feet are glued to the ground.

    "Lifting my feet to put on the slippers is a big task. I always fear falling backwards", says Urmi.

2. Turning:

> Making a turn at any point is one big reason for falls in patients of Parkinson's disease. Making a turn at any point requires a shift in the balance in the body from one part to another. Patients usually take slower steps and find their feet trembling.

How can walking be a solution?

"Put your shoes on!"- Urmi.

Walking has proved to be beneficial in all aspects of our lives, but for the patients suffering from Parkinson's disease, it becomes a game-changer.

"Consistent walking has delayed the symptoms of the disease", says the physiotherapist.

30 minutes of daily walking improves the motor functions and mood by 15%, attention and response by 14% and tiredness and lethargy by 11%. It has shown to improve the gait and balance.

"My gait staggered. I felt anxious when people looked at me. But I had no choice, so I continued. I take support from the walls and stick. It took me 7 months but now I feel confident", says Rama, 68-year-old patient.

> "The neuroplasticity created from exercise in patients with Parkinson's disease may actually outweigh the effects of neurodegeneration"
>
> -Padilla-Davidson.

"Until the time I focused on my gait, it was tough for me to walk. I believed that my walk was fine and walked on paved roads without traffic. I sometimes skipped and jumped too!", said Neerja Das, 33, an engineer suffering from Young Onset Parkinson's Disease (YOPD).

It is observed that patients suffering from YOPD benefit easily from walking rather than the older patients. Most old people who start walking delay other symptoms and complications of the disease.

Gait compensation strategies:

There is no single way that can help in maintaining an independent life with Parkinson's. The stiffness of limbs makes them take smaller steps that lead to falls. Thus, in order to avoid falls, the person should practice taking larger steps. They should walk in broader spaces to prevent freezing. The person should practice breathing exercises to reduce anxiety which is the leading cause of freezing.

The person may also take help of walking aids. In order to prevent falls while turning, the person should turn in wider circles. It is important to make strategic weight shifts before stepping to maintain the required balance.

The patient can also mimic the steps taken by the other person and follow their gait. They can start by focusing on their gait by counting the number of steps they have taken.

Cycling or jumping helps in improving the gait as the legs are used in different ways to move.

Strategies that prevent falls:

1. Allowing the arms to move. The swinging of arms during walking resists a fall.
2. Making the heel strike the ground first. Patients with Parkinson's disease have difficulty in lifting their feet completely hence their toes strike the ground first and that makes them fall.
3. While walking humans shift the complete weight of the body on the legs, one at a time. The patients with Parkinson's shift less weight on their legs hence the balance is not maintained. This can be improved by practicing one leg stand in which the person stands on one leg with another leg up. This helps in improving the weight shift. It also helps in developing steadiness, strength and confidence.
4. The most peculiar feature of the disease is the stooped posture of the patients. Physiotherapist Dr. Doug Weiss suggest backward walking to improve it. According to him, one should take support from a wall or a chair and practice walking backwards for 10 secs and then

turn and repeat the process on the other
side.

5. Sit to stand without taking any support.
    This builds strength and improves
    balance of the body.

> Left. Right. Heel to toe. One foot ahead of other.
> Do this without thought. Easy. Free.

Nordic walking in Parkinson's Disease:

Nordic walking is a form of fitness walking that uses specially designed poles. It is similar to regular walking, but the poles are used to propel the body forward, which engages more muscles and provides a more intense workout.

The arms and legs move in a coordinated rhythm, and the length of the stride is determined by the range of arm movement. A longer pole thrust will result in a longer stride and a more powerful swing of both the arms and the pelvis.

The poles provide the required support and balance that help in maintaining a strong and independent walking pattern. As the poles are pushed backwards with strength, the cardiovascular system is challenged harder and the output increases by 40%.

The pushing action of the poles increases strength of the posture muscles making the person more aware of their posture.

The walking speed is increased, boosting the confidence and the overall balance of the body.

Chapter 9: Daily Strength, Daily Wins: Transforming Parkinson's with strength training

The third stage of Parkinson's disease: It is the stage which is characterized by loss of balance. This takes place due to the reduction in muscle strength. This is an additional motor impairment.

Why muscle contraction becomes difficult?

Gencrally, the lower limbs of the patient lose strength partially due to the inactivity and partly due to the reduction in dopamine. This leads to the overactivity of GABA, a neurotransmitter that alters nerve signalling and alters the ability of the cell to send and receive messages.

GABA blocks messages in the movement centre of the brain. This further leads to alteration in the somatic motor activities resulting in difficulties in the contraction of muscles.

Muscle Strength: It refers to the ability to contract and expand muscles quickly against any resistance. It is the force that moves a door and lifts a weight.

Muscle power: Adding speed to strength gives power. Muscle strength and power helps the body to move safely.

Here's a way to gauge the overall physical capability:

Hand and Grip Strength: Can the patient easily open tight jar lids or twist off bottle caps?

Lower Body Strength: Can the patient participate in playful activities like tug-of-war without undue strain?

Agility and Coordination: Can the patient comfortably adjust your walking speed from slow to fast?

Core and Leg Strength: Can the patient rise from a low chair without using arms for support?

Balance: Can the patient easily get down to the floor and back up, even if they hold onto something for initial stability?

If some of these tasks feel challenging, then strength-training exercises need to be incorporated into the daily routine.

External resistance can be by means of cycle ergometer, weight machine, elastic band, punching bag, and water depending on the stage of the patient. The intensity is increased as the patient starts gaining strength.

How to Develop Stronger Muscles

Here's what to consider for building muscle strength:

Progressive Overload:

- Patient should engage in a physical activity program at least twice a week.
- The intensity of workout should be gradually increased.

This can be achieved by:

- Lifting heavier weights.
- Performing more repetitions or sets of each exercise.
- Shortening rest periods between sets.

Targeting the major muscle Groups:

Focus on exercises that engage the major muscle groups:

- Arms (biceps, triceps, shoulders)
- Legs (quadriceps, hamstrings, calves)
- Trunk (core muscles in the back and abdomen)

Studies have shown that people with mild to moderate Parkinson's disease can safely participate in strength training that uses resistance beyond their own body weight. This type of training has been found to improve both physical abilities and overall well-being in the patients. To further solidify the positive impact of strength training, clinical trials that incorporate specific assessments of muscle strength are needed.

Aerobic Exercises:

Appropriate aerobic exercises include:

Quick step ups: Quick step-up aerobics is a high-energy workout that utilizes a raised platform to target the lower body and cardiovascular system. By repeatedly stepping up and down from the platform, the heart rate gets elevated, leg muscles get strengthened, coordination is improved.

Fast walking: Brisk walking is a fantastic way to reap the benefits of aerobic exercise. It elevates the heart rate and breathing, efficiently burning calories and strengthening the cardiovascular system. This accessible activity requires minimal equipment, just a good pair of shoes, and can be done almost anywhere.

Swimming: Swimming is a particularly well-suited aerobic exercise for individuals with Parkinson's disease. The buoyancy of water provides gentle support for muscles and joints, reducing strain and the risk of falls. This allows for a wider range of motion and more freedom in movement compared to land-based exercises. Additionally, the resistance of water during movement strengthens muscles and improves coordination.

Cycling (Static Bike): It provides a low-impact workout that strengthens muscles, improves cardiovascular health, and enhances coordination. This low-stress activity can also help manage common Parkinson's symptoms like stiffness, tremor, and fatigue. Regular cycling sessions can lead to better balance and increased flexibility, making everyday activities easier.

Research suggests that aerobic exercises can significantly benefit Parkinson's disease patients.

Following the American College[21] of Sports Medicine's recommendation of at least 3 sessions

---

[21] Erwin EH. (2020). *High-Intensity Interval Cycle Ergometer Training in Parkinson's Disease: Protocol for*

per week, lasting 30-60 minutes each, for at least 12 weeks, has shown long-term improvements (beyond 12 weeks) in both motor and cognitive function.

These improvements include better walking speed, increased aerobic capacity, stronger leg muscles, improved attention, and enhanced executive functioning.

Even shorter aerobic exercise programs (3 sessions per week, lasting 30-60 minutes each, for 4 weeks) may lead to some motor function improvements, like faster walking speed and better aerobic capacity.

Lower Limb training[22]:

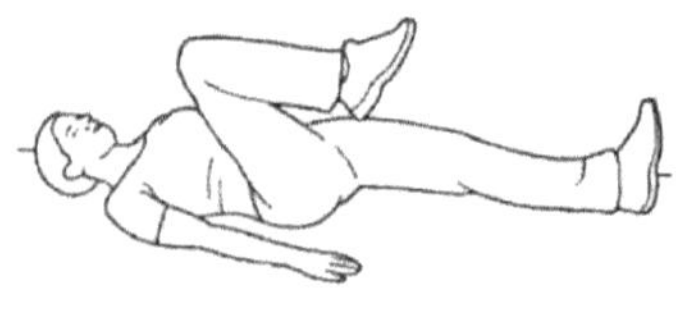

Hip and Knee bends: With slow and controlled movement, lift one leg, keeping the knee bent and pointing towards the ceiling. The leg is gently lowered and then straightened. The process is repeated with the other leg.

Identifying Individual Response Patterns Using a Single-Subject Research Design. Frontiers in Neurology
[22] *Exercise and Advice for People with Parkinson's Disease* NHS Trust

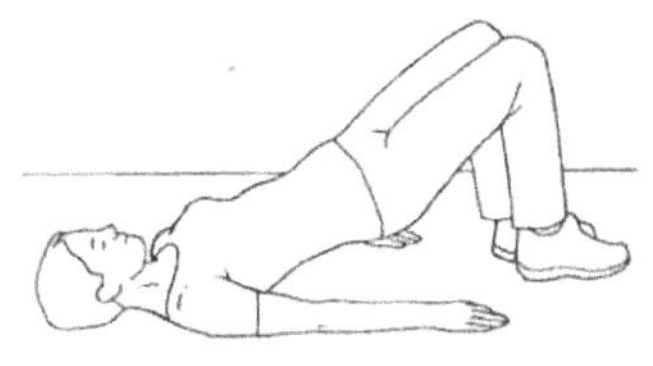

Pelvic Bridging: The patient should assume a lying position with the knees bent, feet flat on the bed, and hip-width apart. Core muscles should be engaged by drawing the navel inwards. The lower back should be pressed against the bed to slowly lift the hips upwards. This bridge position should be held for three seconds.

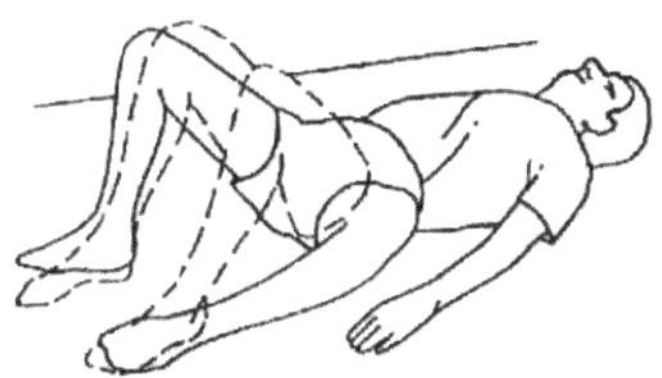

Single Knee drop out: Maintaining the previously described knee bend, one knee should be lowered out to the side in a controlled motion. Then, the should be brought back to the starting position. This exercise is repeated for each leg.

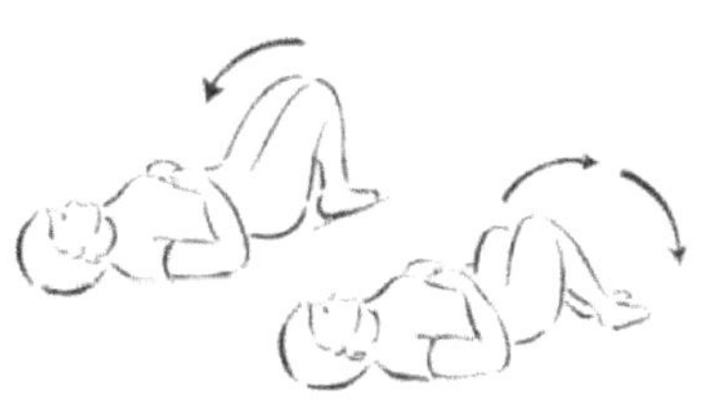

Knee Rolls: Starting position:

The patient should lie on the back with the knees bent and feet flat on the floor.

Movement: Knees are rotated slowly towards the right side, keeping the shoulders flat on the ground. After a brief pause, the starting position is maintained. The same rotation is repeated with towards the left side.

Lower-limb resistance training is a valuable tool for rehabilitating individuals with Parkinson's disease.

Notably, resistance training interventions significantly improved leg strength and quality of life in the patients. While gait performance also showed some improvement, further research is needed to determine the full extent of this benefit.

Safety and Precautions:

The exercise should be discontinued immediately and medical attention should be given to patients if they experience sudden shortness of breath, chest pain, angina, or dizziness.

Doctor should be consulted before starting any new exercise program, especially if the patient hasn't been active for a while.

Mild muscle soreness is common after initial workouts, but this will subside as the muscles adapt.

The intensity and duration of the exercise should be gradually increased over several weeks.

Progress should be tracked on a regular basis.

If there is significant pain, then the exercise should be immediately stopped.

If any discomfort is experienced, the repetitions should be reduced or the exercise should be discontinued.

It should always be remembered that while performing standing exercises, a stable object should always be held for balance.

Chapter 10: Beyond Exercise: Advanced strategies for Parkinson's Management

While medication plays a central role in managing Parkinson's disease, the journey towards optimal well-being often requires a multifaceted approach.

Beyond traditional treatments, advanced strategies have emerged to empower individuals with Parkinson's disease in navigating the complexities of the condition.

These advanced techniques aim to address the spectrum of symptoms, including motor and non-motor challenges thereby making the patients gain control over their lives.

Deep Brain Stimulation therapy

In 1986, in order to overcome these tremors and advanced effects, Deep Brain Stimulation therapy[23] was introduced. Deep Brain Stimulation (DBS) is a surgical procedure that involves implanting electrodes in specific areas of the brain. These electrodes deliver electrical impulses that can help to regulate abnormal activity in the brain and improve symptoms of Parkinson's disease.

For this, the surgeons precisely implant one or more thin wires (called leads or electrodes) into specific areas of the brain during a minimally invasive surgical procedure.

These leads then receive mild electrical stimulation from a small pulse generator that is implanted in the chest.

Continuous pulses of electrical current from the neurostimulator pass through the leads and into the brain.

A few weeks after the neurostimulator has been implanted, the doctor programs it to deliver an electrical signal. This programming process may take multiple visits over a period of weeks or months to ensure that the current is properly adjusted and providing effective results.

In adjusting the device, the doctor seeks an optimal balance between improving symptom control and minimizing side effects.

---

[23] Groiss, Wojtecki, Südmeyer and Schnitzler. (2009). *Deep Brain Stimulation in Parkinson's Disease.* NIH

Proper patient selection, precise placement of the leads, and careful adjustment of the pulse generator are essential for successful DBS surgery.

DBS does not completely resolve the symptoms of Parkinson's disease or other conditions, but it can significantly reduce a patient's need for medications and improve their quality of life.

It proved to be highly effective but still had its drawbacks:

- Firstly, it is a very costly treatment. Hence, not many patients could afford it.
- Secondly, it could be used for idiopathic patients who are below the age of 75 and have achieved 30% improvement with regard to dopamine induced medication.
- Thirdly, it could not be used with patients showing severe psychiatric disorders such as dementia, personality disorders, depressions.
- Finally, it resulted in various neuropsychiatric effects and speech problems. It also resulted in severe complications like intracerebral hemorrhage (simply brain hemorrhage).

Deep Brain stimulation showed marked improvement of motor functions but its effect on the natural course of disease is yet unknown.

Stem Cell Therapy

Stem Cell Therapy originated in 1958 when French Oncologist, Georges Mathe successfully performed the first bone marrow transplantation. By 1998, the scientists had found ways to derive stem cells from human embryos and grow them in the laboratory.

Stem cells are undifferentiated group of cells that have the potential to develop into many different kinds of cells in the body. So, if certain cells get damaged in the body, then stem cells can take up the function of those cells and hence they repair the damage. In the case of Parkinson's disease, the cells that produce dopamine could be generated.

Stem cells were considered to open new pathways for successful treatment of various diseases. However, it was not that easy. The stem cells were derived from the frozen embryos that get destroyed when the new cells are created.

This raised ethical questions and controversies and became a subject of national debate in the United States. The decision was pending on the government as the research could not get the required boost without federal funding.

In 2001, President George W Bush came up with a hard decision. He backed the stem cell research by limiting it only to the use of existing stem cells only. He rejected the use of any new embryos. This became a big obstacle for the new treatment.

In 2009, President Barack Obama signed an Executive order revoking the previous orders allowing federally funded research on hundreds of viable embryonic stem cells.

In 2019, the administration under Donald Trump banned the use of fetal tissues for research.

This limitation was ended by the Joe Biden administration in 2021.

tDCS (transcranial Direct Current Stimulation) application

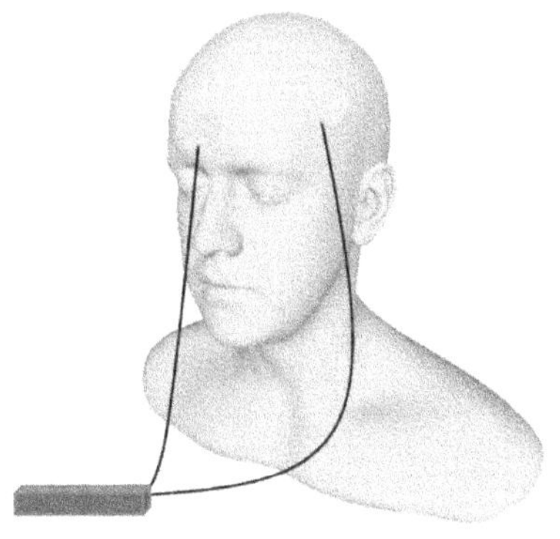

A non-invasive brain stimulation technique known as Transcranial Direct Current Stimulation (tDCS)[24] involves the painless application of a low-intensity electrical current to the scalp via electrodes. This process induces an electric field between an anode and cathode in the brain, altering the resting membrane potential of pre- and post-synaptic neurons

---

[24] Knechtel, L. (2013). *Transcranial direct current stimulation: Neurophysiology and clinical application.* Neuropsychiatry, 3(1), 89-96.

without directly triggering neuronal firing, as seen in electroconvulsive stimulation.

Numerous clinical studies have demonstrated promising effects of tDCS in treating conditions such as depression, chronic pain, schizophrenia, dementia, Parkinson's disease, and cerebral stroke. This technique has the potential to modulate brain region activity and enhance their responsiveness to signals.

Applying a positive current (anodal stimulation) to the motor cortex facilitates the responsiveness of the associated brain cells, whereas a negative current (cathodal stimulation) inhibits their activity.

This modulation can influence the acquisition of new motor skills such as walking, upper limb functions, and functional locomotion, as well as cognitive symptoms in Parkinson's disease.

A systematic review of randomized clinical trials revealed that administering cerebellar tDCS at 4 mA for 20 minutes resulted in immediate improvement in balance following the intervention, although it did not show significant enhancement in gait.

Parkinson's disease is marked by the depletion of dopamine-producing neurons in the substantia nigra. In tDCS, electrodes positioned on the scalp administer a mild electrical current to the head, capable of either stimulating or inhibiting neuronal function and prompting dopamine release.

This method is generally well-received, with minimal adverse effects, typically limited to mild skin irritation at the stimulation site.

Transcranial magnetic stimulation

Repetitive transcranial magnetic stimulation (rTMS) is a technique that uses focused magnetic pulses to target specific areas of the brain. [25]

In this technique patients sit with a large coil placed near their head. This coil generates short bursts of magnetism, creating an electrical current that impacts brain activity in targeted areas. This can lead to changes in the electrical charge of brain cells, potentially producing beneficial effects, as studies have shown.

It's being investigated as a potential treatment for various mental and neurological conditions. It increases the level of dopamine in the brain.[26]

The success of rTMS depends on several factors, including how often and how strong the pulses are, the length of treatment, the targeted area, the number of sessions, and the individual patient's characteristics like age, condition, medications, and specific symptoms.

---

[25] SK Mann. (March 2023). *Repetitive Transcranial Magnetic Stimulation*. NIH
[26] ME Keck. (2002*). Repetitive transcranial magnetic stimulation increases the release of dopamine in the mesolimbic and mesostriatal system.* NIH

Functional electrical stimulation (FES)

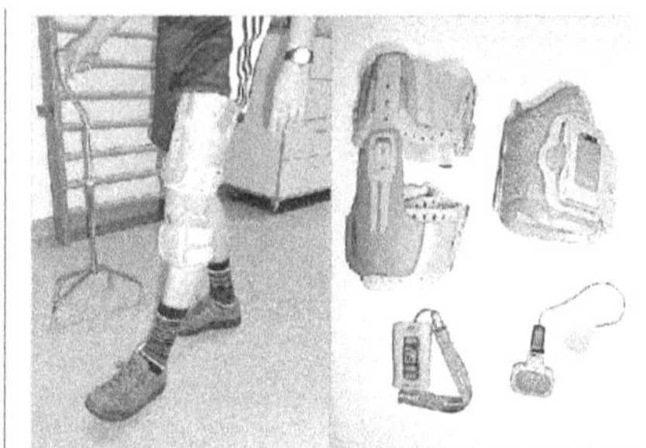

FES, or Functional Electrical Stimulation, employs low-energy electrical signals to activate muscles that are not functioning at their full capacity. This technique involves wearing a compact battery-powered device on the leg to administer FES, aiding in various daily activities. Skin electrodes are positioned over the head of the fibula bone and the tibialis anterior muscle to deliver electrical stimulation to the common peroneal nerve.

In Parkinson's disease, there is a rise in motor-cognitive requirements making tasks like walking while engaging in conversation challenging.[27] Certain research indicates that FES may alleviate symptoms and enhance mobility in Parkinson's disease patients. For instance, a feasibility study demonstrated that FES enhanced both gait and upper limb function in a group of 11 individuals with Parkinson's disease. Additionally, another study suggests that FES-assisted cycling can

---

[27] McIsaac, Tara L., et al. *Cognitive-Motor Interference in Neurodegenerative Disease: A Narrative Review and Implications for Clinical Management.* Frontiers in Psychology, vol. 9, 2018, pp. 1551.

enable individuals with Parkinson's disease to pedal at a quicker and smoother pace.

FES helps in various ways, including:

- Alleviating muscle spasms
- Preventing or delaying disuse atrophy
- Enhancing local blood circulation
- Facilitating muscle re-education
- Sustaining or enhancing range of motion

Cranial Electrotherapy Stimulation

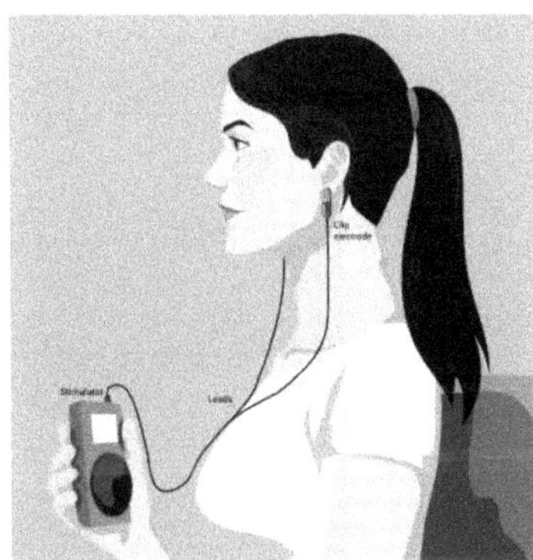

CES uses a very weak electrical current, like a tiny tickle, to stimulate the brain. Most people don't even feel it, but it's strong enough to have an effect.

It uses a device that transmit electricity to the brain.

he device influences brain activity in two important ways. First, it stimulates nerves in the head and neck, including the vagus nerve, which is involved in many bodily functions. Second, directly modulating cortical oscillations in the temporal lobe, which is part of the default mode network.

Chapter 11: Demystifying Parkinson's Disease: Navigating the Maze of Parkinson's Myths

There are many misconceptions surrounding Parkinson's disease. Some people think it's just a disorder that causes tremors or that it's a death sentence. However, the truth is more complex. Parkinson's disease can impact people in different ways, and there have been significant advances in managing its symptoms.

Myth: Parkinson's disease is just a motor condition.

Reality: Parkinson's disease is often characterized by tremors, muscle rigidity, slowness of movement, and a masked facial expression. However, this neurological condition encompasses a much broader spectrum of symptoms.

Increasing recognition is being given to non-motor symptoms, which can significantly impact a patient's life. These include cognitive decline, anxiety, depression, fatigue, sleep disturbances, and more. In some cases, non-motor symptoms can be even more debilitating than the well-known motor issues targeted by traditional treatments.

Myth: Parkinson's medications can have side effects that mimic Parkinson's symptoms.

Reality: The misconception that Parkinson's disease medications are toxic and accelerate the condition persists, despite being thoroughly debunked. Levodopa, the mainstay of Parkinson's treatment, is a powerful medication that significantly improves motor symptoms. However, a persistent myth suggests that Levodopa hastens the disease progression. This misconception portrays Levodopa as somehow a poisonous and detrimental remedy to patients in the long run. Extensive clinical research conducted over the decades definitively refuted this misconception. The study demonstrated that patients receiving Levodopa experienced no worsening condition compared to those given a placebo. In fact, Levodopa demonstrably improved their condition by the study's conclusion. Crucially, Levodopa has not been shown to be toxic.

Myth: Everyone faces tremors.

Reality: Tremor is a hallmark symptom of Parkinson's disease, yet it isn't universally present. Intriguingly, some patients experience non-motor symptoms before tremor manifests.

Furthermore, roughly 20% of individuals with Parkinson's disease never develop a tremor.

The reasons behind this variability remain elusive, but researchers believe the severity and presence of tremor may be linked to the specific brain regions affected by the disease.

Myth: There is no other alternative beyond drugs.

Reality: A common misconception persists that medication is the sole approach to manage Parkinson's symptoms and progression. However, a growing body of evidence suggests otherwise.

Staying physically active plays a significant role in mitigating symptoms and potentially slowing disease progression. Research demonstrates that individuals who initiate exercise earlier and maintain a minimum of 2.5 hours weekly experience a slower decline in quality of life compared to those who begin later. Therefore, establishing regular exercise habits from the outset is crucial for overall disease management.

The impact of exercise extends beyond just motor symptoms. Studies have revealed its effectiveness in improving sleep problems commonly associated with Parkinson's disease.

Myth: People with Parkinson's disease may experience periods of worsened symptoms.

Reality: Unlike conditions like multiple sclerosis that exhibit symptom flare-ups, Parkinson's disease typically presents with a gradual progression of symptoms. These symptoms may fluctuate throughout the day, but overall, worsen slowly.

A sudden worsening of symptoms in Parkinson's disease patients often points to other underlying causes.

According to studies, infections are the most frequent culprit, responsible for over a quarter (25.6%) of these exacerbations. Other contributing factors may include anxiety, medication errors or non-adherence, medication side effects, and post-surgical health decline. It is also reported that most of these episodes stem from reversible or treatable causes.

Myth: The treatment for Parkinson's is only effective only during the initial stages.

Reality: While Parkinson's disease remains incurable, medications like Levodopa offer significant symptom management. Levodopa is converted into dopamine by the body, replenishing the crucial neurotransmitter lost in Parkinson's patients.

A persistent misconception suggests Levodopa's effectiveness wanes after five years. Fortunately, this is untrue. Levodopa can provide relief for decades, although its potency may gradually decrease over time.

However, it's true that over time, individual Levodopa doses may provide symptom relief for shorter periods. This "wearing-off" phenomenon signifies the return of symptoms before the next scheduled dose.

Myth: Parkinson's disease is a life-threatening condition.

Reality: While a Parkinson's disease diagnosis can be life-altering, it's important to dispel the misconception that it's a terminal illness. Unlike strokes or heart attacks, Parkinson's disease itself isn't directly fatal. However, the quality of care, encompassing both medical support and self-management, significantly impacts well-being.

As the disease progresses, the risk of falls increases, which can lead to serious complications. This underscores the importance of exercise and physical therapy in maintaining mobility.

Another concern is the increased susceptibility to infections in later stages. Difficulty recognizing early signs of infection can lead to delayed treatment and potentially serious consequences. Regular medical check-ups become even more crucial in this context.

This rewrite uses a more positive and empowering tone. It clarifies the distinction between Parkinson's and fatal conditions and emphasizes the role of proactive management in living well with the disease.

Myth: Deep brain stimulation is an experimental therapy.

Reality: Deep brain stimulation, or DBS, is a surgical procedure for Parkinson's disease that targets specific areas of the brain responsible for movement control. It is typically considered when medications become less effective in managing motor symptoms like tremors, stiffness, and slowness of movement.

While DBS might seem like a cutting-edge procedure, it has actually been a well-established and successful treatment for decades. Similar to a pacemaker for the heart, DBS uses implanted electrodes to deliver electrical pulses to specific brain regions, helping to regulate abnormal activity and improve movement control. Over the decades, DBS has become a standard treatment option for carefully selected patients with Parkinson's disease.

"Never give up on yourself." - Muhammad Ali

Dr. Rajat Gupta(PT): A Multifaceted Approach to Wellness (Dehradun, India)

Dr. Rajat Gupta is a leading healthcare professional in Dehradun, India, with over 10 years of experience in Osteopathy, Chiropractic care, and Physiotherapy. This comprehensive approach allows him to provide patients with a holistic range of treatments for musculoskeletal conditions and pain management.

Instagram: www.instagram.com/rajatgupta2063

Email: Rajat2063@gmail.com
Facebook: www.facebook.com/rajatgupta2063

Suravi Sharan, a captivating writer based in India, has a unique, fiery style of putting light on issues of daily life in an unapologetic manner. She is passionate about crafting clear and informative content on health (physical and mental) and wellness topics. She is also an academician who enjoys shaping young minds with her liberated thoughts.

Instagram: SURAVI SHARAN (@adisaranaa)

Email: suravi2410@gmail.com

Facebook:
www.facebook.com/profile.php?id=1000920398
11968

More from Suravi Sharan

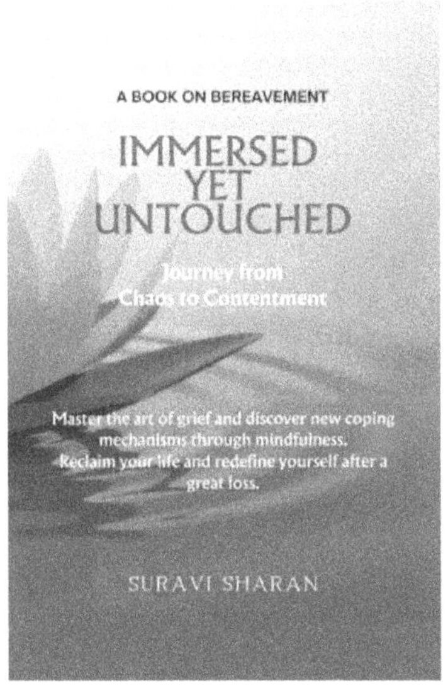

How does it feel like, what it teaches, and how to live with it- without losing ourselves?

Losing a loved one is one of the most difficult experiences a person can go through. It can be hard to know how to cope with the pain of grief, and it can be easy to feel like you're all alone.

If you're struggling to cope with the loss of a loved one, this book can help. It provides the information and support you need to start your journey to better healing.

Link to buy: https://amzn.in/d/fV5uNoQ

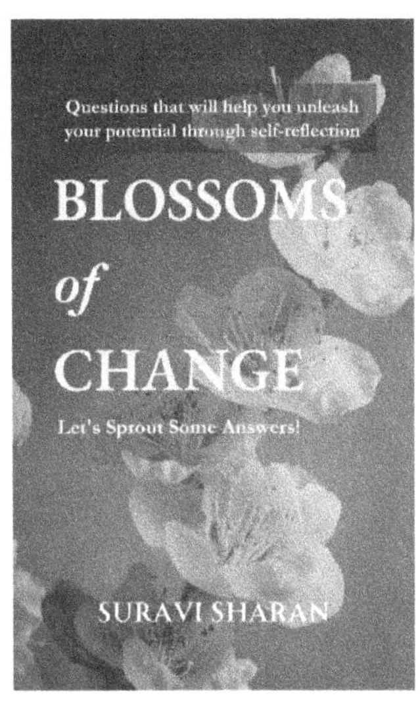

Do you yearn to break free from limitations and live life to its fullest?

This book invites you into a conversation that will prompt you to sprout answers about narratives from your everyday life, by being your companion, and an angel on your shoulder.

It ignites a journey of self-discovery through powerful questions designed to unlock your hidden potential.

Stop settling for the ordinary.

Become the best version of yourself.

Are you ready to unlock your potential?

Start your journey today!

Link to buy: https://amzn.in/d/ewaP1BS